D1493616

Healthy Smoke

350 Diffuser Recipes for a Healthy Mind, Body and Soul

Rica V. Gadi

Copyright © 2018 by The Oil Natural Empress

All rights reserved. This book or any portion thereof may not be reproduced or used in any manner whatsoever without the express written permission of the publisher except for the use of brief quotations in a book review.

Printed in the United States of America

First Printing, 2018

ISBN-13: 9781982984816

http://oilnaturalempress.com/

DISCLAIMER: This document is a compilation of recipes used successfully by EO enthusiasts who use only high-quality, therapeutic-grade essential oils as determined by many factors including growth, growth location, harvesting process, distillation method used, etc. Please be advised that not all essential oils are created equally, and not all essential oils are suitable for topical use or ingestion. Please do your research before choosing the brand(s) of essential oils you decide to use as well as supplies you use. Always follow label directions on the essential oil bottles.

All the recipes in this book have been inspired by essential oil believers. However, we are not medical practitioners and cannot diagnose, treat or prescribe treatment for any health condition or disease. Just a precaution, before using any alternative medicines, natural supplements, or vitamins, you should always discuss the products you are using or intend to use with your doctor, especially if you are pregnant, trying to get pregnant or nursing.

All information contained within this book is for reference purposes only, and is not intended to substitute advice given by a pharmacist, physician or other licensed health-care professional. As such, the author is not responsible for any loss, claim or damage arising from use of the essential oil recipes contained herein.

This book is dedicated to all the strong people who are taking responsibility of your own well being and doing something to be better.

All my heartfelt gratitude to the following people: my mom Ruby Jane, you have made me everything I am today; my dad Nestor-- my eternal, my angel, and the source of my perseverance; Mommyling, my spiritual guide ; Ria & Joe, the true witnesses of my transformation and my foundation pillars; Ellie Jane, the sparkle of our eyes;

Juan, thanks for always encouraging me to push harder - you are my ONE; Rocco & Radha, my reason for everything.

The Love of my family and friends is the fountain of inspiration that never runs dry. Thank you for constantly inspiring me, motivating me, and loving me unconditionally.

This book will never be complete without the help of my trusted and talented friends: Golda, Jessica, Lika and BFFs at NOW for the moral support.

Diffusers for Essential Oils is the safest method to enjoy EOs without the risk of an allergic reaction.

When the "Oil Recipe Bible" came out, people started to ask me about recipes only for diffusers

This is why I decided to put together this Diffusers for Essential Oils recipe book. All the recipes in this book are all for diffusing.

Remember this is a diffusing recipe book and should not be used for any blends like rollers, sprays and scrubs as those will use a different dilution than the ones for diffusing.

Enjoy, and I am sure in a matter of time, your oil diffusing habit will be a more permanent part of your days, if it isn't already. Happy Blending :)

Table of Contents

Diffusing Essential Oils
Some Tidbits You Need To Know

Our sense of smell is one of our most powerful senses, and as you have noticed in your own experience that some scents affect your more positively in your minds than others. The body contains over 1,000 receptors for smell—way more receptors than for any of our other senses.

Diffusion Essential Oils means the process vaporizes oils into air by releasing tiny amounts into the air. Inhalation is totally safe and is super low risk. Chances of any EO rising to dangerous levels while diffusion is slim to none.

Diffusing Essential Oils around newborns, babies, young children, pregnant or nursing women, and pets should be done with caution. Read up on safety.

It is advisable that Diffusing Essential Oils for only about 30–45 minutes at a time to be most effective. NEVER leave your diffuser on overnight. Make sure your diffuser is filled with the right amount of water and you understand the operating directions.

While diffusing essential oils, be sure that your space has great ventilation. Crack a window open if the scent become to strong.

Never add Carrier Oils to your diffuser. This may cause your diffuser to malfunction. Clean your diffuser at least 3 times a week with warm water and natural soap to ensure the diffuser is well maintained and bacteria and mold does not accumulate.

It is not advisable to use EO in humidifiers. These are not made to release EOS

Diffusing Essential Oils Basic Guidelines

Just a few things you need to know and prepare before getting started Diffusing Essential Oils.

Things you need:
Ultrasonic Oil Diffuser
Essential Oils
Water

Just follow the number of drops in the recipe, drop on to an oil diffuser and fill the rest with water.

All diffusers are different and will have its own water minimum and maximum level. Read the diffuser instruction before use.

Ideally, it is best to diffuse for 15-30 minutes and turn off the diffuser. The effect should be good for at least 2-3 hours. Turn your diffuser back on after 3 hours to reinforce oil diffusing effects.

Diffusing Blends Recipes

Air Purifier

Fresh Citrus
1-2 Drops each of
Lemon
Lime
Wild Orange
Grapefruit
Bergamot

Shoo Germs
4 Drops Shield
2 Drops Lemon
1 Drop Melaleuca

Clean Fresh Air
4 RC
2 Purification

So Fresh & So Clean
5 RC
5 Lemon

Purify Fresh
3 Purification
3 Thieves

Pure Delight
1-2 Drops Lemongrass
5 Drops Tea Tree
4 Drops Clove Bud

Fantastic Fresh
3 Peppermint
5 Purification

Mighty Air Clean
4 Drops Immune Aid
4 Drops Germ Fighter

Pure Air Supply
1 Drop Thyme
3 Drop Eucalyptus
6 Drops Lemon

Freakishly Clean
1 Drop Cinnamon Bark
3 Drops Fresh Ginger
6 Drops Sweet Orange

Allergy Relief

Allergy Buster
3 Drops Peppermint
3 Drops Lavender
3 Drops Lemon

Allergy Ally
2 Lavender
2 Lemon
2 Peppermint (+ 2 Melaleuca, optional)

Shoo Achoo
5 Drops Lavender
3 Drops Vetiver
2 Drops Ylang Ylang

Stuffed Up No More
3 Drops Peppermint
2 Drops Eucalyptus
2 Drops Tea Tree
1 Drop Lemon

Sneeze Be Gone
3 Drops Peppermint
3 Drops Lemon
3 Drops Eucalyptus

AntiBac Mix
3 Drops Tea Tree
2 Drops Lavender
2 Drops Peppermint

Sinusitis Helper
4 Drops Lavender
4 Drops Peppermint
2 Drops Frankincense
2 Drops Basil

Allergy Tamer
3 Drops Eucalyptus
3 Drops Peppermint
3 Drops Rosemary

Anxiety

Stress No More
5 Drops Sandalwood
1 Drop Neroli
1 Drop Roman Chamomile
1 Drop Lavender

Break Free
4 Drops Lavender
2 Drops Lemon
2 Drops Ylang Ylang

Chill Pill
3 Drops Orange
2 Drops Bergamot
2 Drops Lavender

Shake It Off
3 Drops Frankincense
2 Drops Lavender
2 Drops Wild Orange

Harmony Delight
3 Drops Patchouli
2 Drops White Fir
2 Drops Lavender

Fidget Fighter
4 Drops Lavender
2 Drops Rosemary

No Worries Dear
3 Drops Patchouli
3 Drops Bergamot

Let Go and Unwind
2 Drops Geranium
2 Drops Clary Sage
1 Drop Patchouli
1 Drop Ylang Ylang

Anxiety Tamer
2 Drops Cedarwood
2 Drops Wild Orange
1 Drop Ylang Ylang
1 Drop Patchouli

Aroma

Hello There
3 Drops Lavender
3 Drops Lemon
3 Drops Rosemary

Wonderful Day
3 Drops Wild Orange
3 Drops Grapefruit
2 Drops Lemon
2 Drop Bergamot

So Fresh So Clear
3 Drops Melaleuca
3 Drops Lemon
3 Drops Lime

Fresh Breeze
4 Drops Purify
4 Drops Lemon

Air So Fresh
4 Drops Vetiver
3 Drops Lemon
3 Drops Peppermint

Air Delight
3 Drops Lemon
2 Drops Melaleuca
2 Drops Cilantro
2 Drops Lime

Clean Fresh Scents
3 Drops Lemon
2 Drops Melaleuca
2 Drops Lime
2 Drops White Fir
2 Drops Cilantro

Gentleman's Breeze
3 Drops Bergamot
3 Drops Cypress
3 Drops Arborvitae

The Man Cave Aroma
2 Drops White Fir
2 Drops Cypress
2 Drops Wintergreen

Fall Mist
4 Drops Wild Orange
3 Drops Cinnamon
3 Drops Ginger

Summer Breeze
3 Drops Grapefruit
3 Drops Lavender
2 Drops Lemon
2 Drops Spearmint

Springtime Madness
2 Drops Geranium
3 Drops Lavender
3 Drops Roman Chamomile

Winter Wonders
3 Drops White Fir
3 Drops Wild Frange
2 Drops Wintergreen

Holiday Cheer
4 Drops Patchouli
4 Drops Cinnamon
3 Drops Orange
2 Drops Clove
1 Drop Ylang Ylang

Spicy Chai Mix
3 Drops Cardamom
2 Drops Cassia
2 Drops Clove
1 Drop Ginger

Citrus and Spice
4 Drops Wild Orange
3 Drops Cinnamon
2 Drops Clove

The Candy Shop
4 Drops Wild Orange
4 Drops Wintergreen

Woodsy Fresh
4 Drops Frankincense
3 Drops White Fir
2 Drops Cedarwood

Citrus Outdoors
2 Drops Lime
2 Drops Lemon
1 Drop Orange
1 Drop Bergamot
1 Drop White Fir

Sweet Fresh & Spicy
4 Drops Wild Orange
3 Drops Cinnamon
3 Drops Ginger

Odor Buster
5 Drops Lemon
5 Drops Purification

To The Beach We Go
2 Drops Lemon
3 Drops Stress Away

Sun Shiny Day
2 Drops Bergamot
4 Drops Orange
2 Drops Ylang Ylang

Spring Fresh
4 Drops Lavender
4 Drops Orange
2 Drops Geranium

Refresh Seasons
2 Drops Cinnamon Bark
2 Drops Nutmeg
2 Drops Clove

Mrs Claus' Fave
4 Drops Christmas Spirit
4 Drops Stress Away

Happy Citrus
1 Drop Bergamont
1 Drop Grapefruit
1 Drop Lemon
1 Drop Lime
1 Drop Orange

Fresh Rain
4 Drops Lemon
3 Drops Vetiver

Fresh Citrus Vibe
2 Drops Lavender
2 Drops Grapefruit
2 Drops Lemon
2 Drops Peppermint

Feel like a kid again
3 Drops PanAway
3 Drops Stress Away

Skip and Giddy
3 Drops Rosemary
3 Drops Lemon

Lemony Dew
3 Drops Lemongrass
3 Drops Orange

Perky Pumpkin
3 Drops Thieves
3 Drops Orange

Cider Refresh
2 Drops Cinnamon
4 Drops Orange
2 Drops Ginger

Spirit of Christmas
2 Drops Idaho Blue Spruce
2 Drops Idaho Balsam Fir
2 Drops Pine

Good Morning
5 Drops Sweet Orange
5 Drops Grapefruit
2 Drops Lime

For Men
4 Drops Wintergreen
3 Drops Cypress
2 Drops Fir Needle

Autumn Blend
4 Drops Sweet Orange
4 Drops Cassia

Fun Scent
6 Drops Sweet Orange
1 Drop Patchouli
1 Drop Ginger

On A Holiday
2 Drops Fir Needle
2 Drops Cassia
2 Drops Sweet Orange

Squeaky Clean
2 Drops Lavender
2 Drops Lemon
2 Drops Rosemary

Odor no more
2 Drops Lemon
1 Drop Melaleuca
1 Drop Cilantro
1 Drop Lime

Pump up Lemon
1 Drop Lemon
2 Drops Wild Orange
1 Drop Lime
1 Drop Grapefruit

Garden Essentials
1 Drop Geranium
2 Drops Lavender
2 Drops Roman Chamomile

Made for Men
2 Drops White First
2 Drops Cypress
2 Drops Wintergreen

Chill Chai
3 Drops Cardamom
2 Drops Cassia
2 Drops Clove
1 Drop Ginger

Chill Citrus
3 Drops Wild Orange
2 Drops Cinnamon Bark
1 Drop Clove

Walk in the Woods
3 Drops Frankincense
2 Drops White Fir
1 Drop Cedarwood

Sweet Candy Store
2 Drops Wild Orange
2 Drop Wintergreen

Holiday Special
2 Drops White Fir
2 Drops Wild Orange
1 Drop Wintergreen

Dirty no more!
2 Drops Purify Cleansing Blend
4 Drops Lemon
2 Drops Lemon
2 Drops Lime
1 Drop Melaleuca

School Buddy
3 Drops Melaleuca
2 Drops Lemon

No Stink Magic

4 Drops Purification
1 Drop Lemon
1 Drop Melaleuca Alternifolia {Tea Tree}

Mountain Breeze

3 Drops Idaho Balsam Fir
3 Drops Ylang Ylang

Happy Blends

3 Drops Bergamot
2 Drops Grapefruit
1 Drop Ylang Ylang

Hello to New

3 Drops Chamomile
3 Drops Geranium
3 Drops Lavender

Misty Rain

3 Drops Vetiver
3 Drops Lemon

No Itch Blend

3 Drops Lavender
3 Drops Peppermint
3 Drops Lemon

Beach Please
4 Drops Bergamot
4 Drops Lime

Welcome to the Woods
3 Drops White Fir
2 Drops Cedarwood
1 Drop Peppermint
1 Drop Clove

Garden Pleasure
3 Drops Coriander
3 Drops Geranium
2 Drops Orange

Spring treat
4 Drops Orange
4 Drops Ylang Ylang

Awake

Wake Up Happy
4 Drops Wild Orange
4 Drops Peppermint

Jump Out of Bed
4 Drops Lemon
3 Drops Peppermint

Roll Me Up a Great Day
3 Drops Joy
4 Drops Lemon

Sunshine and Motivation
3 Drops Bergamot
3 Drops Ylang Ylang

Brekky and Awesome
2 Drops Black Pepper
2 Drops Orange
1 Drop Cinnamon

Let Your Light Shine Through
2 Drops Juniper Berry
2 Drops Grapefruit
1 Drop Orange

Open the Day Right
2 Drops Frankincense
2 Drops White Fir
1 Drop Black Pepper
1 Drop Bergamot

Easy Morning
2 Drops Lavender
1 Drops Cypress
2 Drops Bergamot
3 Drops Clary Sage

Sunshine Sparkle
2 Drops Peppermint
2 Drops Lime
2 Drops Orange

Make this Day Count
3 Drops Bergamot
2 Drops Frankincense
2 Drops Orange

The New Season
3 Drops Peppermint
2 Drops Lemon
2 Drops Orange

Breathe Easy

Minty Solace
2 Drops Eucalyptus
1 Drop Lemon
2 Drops Peppermint

Health Blend
4 Drops Eucalyptus
4 Drops Peppermint

State of Elevation
2 Drops RC
2 Drops Peppermint

Relaxing Breath
5 Drops Eucalyptus
2 Drops Lemon

Deep Breath Blends
2 Drops Lemon
2 Drops Lavender
2 Drops Peppermint

Clarity and Life
4 Drops Frankincense
3 Drops RC or Eucalyptus

Cough no more!
6 Drops Clary Sage
4 Drops Fir Needle
3 Drops Lavender

Relax and Breathe
1 Drop Bergamot
1 Drop Patchouli
1 Drop Ylang Ylang

Calm and Easy
2 Drops Lemon
2 Drops Eucalyptus
2 Drops Rosemary
1 Drops Thyme

Take a Breath and Slow Down
1 Drops Lavender
2 Drops Peppermint
2 Drops Thyme
3 Drops Eucalyptus

Calming

Good and Calm Blend
2 Drops Rosemary
2 Drops Pine
2 Drops Marjoram
1 Drop Lemon

Don't Worry
3 Drops Lavender
3 Drops Geranium
2 Drops Roman Chamomile
2 Drops Clary Sage
2 Drops Ylang Ylang

Don't Hurry
3 Drops Lavender
3 Drops Lime
3 Drops Mandarin

Keep Calm
4 Drops Lavender
2 Drops Cedarwood
2 Drops Wild Orange
1 Drop Ylang Ylang

Peace and Clarity
3 Drops Frankincense
2 Drops Copaiba

Tension begone!
3 Drops Lavender
2 Drops Stress Away
2 Drops Frankincense

Focus on Easy
5 Drops Frankincense
5 Drops Stress Away

Create Your Own Calm
3 Drops Peppermint
5 Drops Lavender
2 Drops Stress Away

Meditation and Relaxation
4 Drops Bergamot
5 Drops Frankincense

Calm Within
4 Drops Stress Away
4 Drops Orange

Transcend
2 Drops Purification
3 Drops Lemon
3 Drops Orange

Finding Peace
2 Drops Grapefruit
2 Drops Bergamot
2 Drops Lime
2 Drops Ginger
1 Drop Sandalwood

Zen Zoned
3 Drops Orange
3 Drops Patchouli

Tranquil Spirit
2 Drops Lavender
2 Drops Cedarwood
2 Drops Roman Chamomile

Serenity
4 Drops Lavender
3 Drops Geranium
2 Drops Roman Chamomile
2 Drops Clary Sage
2 Drops Ylang Ylang

Peace After the Storm
4 Drops Lavender
3 Drops Chamomile

Quiet Repose
2 Drops Vetiver
2 Drops Cedarwood

Quiescent
2 Drops Grounding Blend
2 Drops Lavender

Quiescent Spirit
1 Drop Lavender
1 Drop Sweet (Wild) Orange
1 Drop Cedarwood
1 Drop Frankincense

After the TurmOil is Peace
2 Drops Lavender
2 Drops Lime
1 Drop Spearmint

Congestion

Chest-Abate
3 Drops Lemon
3 Drops Scotch Pine
3 Drops Lavender
1 Drop Peppermint

Decongestion Blend
3 Drops Juniper Berry
4 Drops Rosemary
4 Drops Frankincense

Chest and Refresh!
4 Drops Cypress
6 Drops Grapefruit

Soothe & Smooth
5 Drops Cedarwood
4 Drops Lavender
1 Drop Chamomile
1 Drop Eucalyptus (optional)

Refresh
5-7 Drops Pine or Cedarwood
5-7 Drops Lavender
4 Drops Eucalyptus
1 Drop Lemon

Full of Life
3-5 Drops Rosemary
2 Drops Thyme
1 Drop Peppermint

Rest and Respire
3 Drops Peppermint
3 Drops Lemon
3 Drops Eucalyptus

Cough no more
2 Drops Oregano
2 Drops Tea Tree
2 Drops Peppermint
2 Drops Lavender
2 Drops Lemon

Breathe in Delight
3 Drops Tea Tree
2 Drops Lavender
2 Drops Peppermint

No More Sniffles
4 Drops Lavender
4 Drops Peppermint
2 Drops Frankincense
2 Drops Basil

Bye Congestion
3 Drops Eucalyptus
3 Drops Peppermint
3 Drops Rosemary

Cough & Colds

Throat Coat
2 Drops Clove
2 Drops Lemon
2 Drops Cinnamon
2 Drops Eucalyptus
2 Drops Rosemary

Cough & Cold Cleanse
3 Drops Rosemary
2 Drops Eucalyptus
2 Drops Peppermint
1 Drops Cypress
1 Drops Lemon

Respiratory Healer
2 Drops Lemon
1 Drops Lime
2 Drops Peppermint
1 Drops Rosemary
2 Drops Eucalyptus
1 Drops Clove

Decongest and Relax
3 Drops RC
3 Drops Lemon
3 Drops Purification

Decongestion Blend
2 Drops Eucalyptus
1 Drops Peppermint
3 Drops Frankincense

Achoo be gone!
4 Drops Thieves
3 Drops Eucalyptus Radiata
3 Drops Lavender

Cure for the Winter Sniffles
1 Drop Lemon
1 Drop Eucalyptus
2 Drops Peppermint
1 Drop Rosemary

Inhale and Exhale Easy
1 Drop Rosemary
2 Drops Eucalyptus
2 Drops Lime
1 Drop Peppermint
1 Drops Frankincense

Breathe Normally
2 Drops Frankincense
2 Drops Orange
1 Drop Eucalyptus

No More Raspy Throat
2 Drops Oregano
2 Drops Rosemary
2 Drops Peppermint
2 Drops Eucalyptus

Cold alleviation
3 Drops Eucalyptus
2 Drops Lavender
2 Drop Peppermint

Colds Begone
3 Drops Eucalyptus
3 Drops Tea Tree

Throat Relief
4 Drops Eucalyptus
2 Drops Myrrh
4 Drops Cedarwood

Body Relief
4 Drops Eucalyptus
2 Drops Ginger
4 Drops Rosemary

Smooth Throat Relief
4 Drops Tea Tree
4 Drops Eucalyptus

Emotional Stability

Worry Free Morning
3 Drops Spearmint
2 Drops Tangerine

Morning Charm
4 Drops Grapefruit
3 Drops Fennel

Morningspiration
2 Drops Lavender
2 Drops Wild Orange
2 Drops Wintergreen
2 Drops White Fir

Harmony Blend
3 Drops Neroli
3 Drops Sweet Orange
1 Drop Frankincense
1 Drop Lemon
1 Drop Ylang Ylang

Tranquil Heart
2 Drops Wild Orange
2 Drops Bergamot
2 Drops Cypress
2 Drops Frankincense

Harmony and Peace
3 Drops Lavender
3 Drops Bergamot

Abounding Peace
3 Drops Peppermint
3 Drops Lemon
2 Drops Orange

Temperate Indulgence
4 Drops Lavender
2 Drops Lemon
2 Drops Ylang Ylang

Quiet Joy
4 Drops Lavender
3 Drops Chamomile

Luminous Tranquility
2 Drops Frankincense
2 Drops Bergamot
2 Drops Orange

Clarity of the Mind
3 Drops Bergamot
2 Drops Lavender
2 Drops Clary Sage
1 Drop Ylang Ylang

Serenity Power
4 Drops Lavender
2 Drops Vetiver

Calm in Chaos

4 Drops Orange
2 Drops Lavender
1 Drop Ylang Ylang

Breathe me happy!
3 Drops Rosemary
3 Drops Peppermint
3 Drops Lemon

Joy Aplenty
2 Drops Grapefruit
3 Drops Peppermint
3 Drops Rosemary

Energy

Joy Overdrive
3 Drops Wild Orange
3 Drops Frankincense
2 Drops Cinnamon

Happiness Madness
3 Drops Grapefruit
3 Drops Joy

Ready for the World
3 Drops Stress Away
3 Drops Peppermint

Born to Crunch It
4 Drops Peppermint
5 Drops Sweet Orange

Motivation on Overdrive
5 Drops Rosemary
5 Drops Grapefruit
5 Drops Lime

Amped!
3 Drops Sweet Orange
3 Drops Grapefruit
2 Drops Lemon
1 Drop Bergamot

Energy Bounty
3 Drops Peppermint
3 Drops Lemon
2 Drops Orange

Energy Treasure
2 Drops Wild Orange
2 Drops Frankincense
2 Drops Cinnamon

Commitment Blend
2 Drops Eucalyptus
2 Drops Geranium
1 Drop Lemon
1 Drop Thyme

Aim Higher
3 Drops Rosemary
2 Drops Lemon
2 Drops Peppermint

Swift Like Bugatti
3 Drops Eucalyptus
2 Drops Lemon
1 Drop Peppermint

North American X-15
3 Drops Orange
2 Drops Lemon
1 Drop Peppermint

Motivate Me Booster
3 Drops Eucalyptus
3 Drops Rosemary

Bullish and Ready
3 Drops White Fir
3 Drops Orange

Speed Racer
4 Drops Peppermint
3 Drops Geranium

Victory Mist
3 Drops Rosemary
2 Drops Peppermint
1 Drop Basil

Make this Day Yours
3 Drops Grapefruit
2 Drops Peppermint
1 Drop Spearmint

Pick Me Up X 12
1 Drop Cardamom
1 Drop Sandalwood
1 Drop Cassia
1 Drop Ginger

Wonder Dose
1 Drop Black Pepper
1 Drop Lime
1 Drop Sweet (Wild) Orange
1 Drop Frankincense

Pumped and Hyped
1 Drop Lime
1 Drop Grapefruit
1 Drop Tangerine
1 Drop Spearmint

Fatigue

Warrior Wonder
2 Drops Juniper Berry
2 Drops Orange
1 Drop Lemon
1 Drop White Fir

Tough Made Easy
2 Drops Eucalyptus
2 Drops Geranium
1 Drop Lemon
1 Drop Thyme

Frisk Away
1 Drops Roman Chamomile
3 Drops Lavender
4 Drops Sandalwood
3 Drops Lemon

Get Moving
5 Drops Lavender
2 Drops Cedarwood
2 Drops Vetiver
2 Drops Patchouli

Sprint in 12
3 Drops Orange
2 Drops Lemon
1 Drop Peppermint

Sprint Runner
3 Drops Rosemary
2 Drops Peppermint
1 Drop Basil

Direct Energy Booster
2 Drops Sandalwood
2 Drops Frankincense
2 Drops Bergamot

War Zone Blend
4 Drops Peppermint
3 Drops Geranium

Power Burst
3 Drops Eucalyptus
3 Drops Rosemary

Trail Blazer
3 Drops White Fir
3 Drops Orange

Focus

Clarity Point
1 Drop Basil
1 Drop Rosemary
2 Drops Lemon
2 Drops Peppermint
2 Drops Grapefruit
2 Drops Lavender

Goal Setter Getter
2 Drops Motivation
1 Drops Tangerine
1 Drops Energy Boost
1 Drops Tangerine
1 Drops Spearmint
1 Drops Lemongrass

Worry Free Clarity
1 Drops Wild Orange
1 Drops Peppermint
1 Drops Rosemary
4 In Tune Focus Blend

Target Shooter
2 Drops Lemon
1 Drop Basil
1 Drop Rosemary
1 Drop Cypress

Study Buddy
3 Drops Lime
3 Drops Rosemary
1 Drop Basil
1 Drop Ginger

Focus Point
2 Drops Frankincense
2 Drops Vetiver
4 Drops Balance

Zero In Factor
2 Drops Peppermint
2 Drops Cinnamon
1 Drop Rosemary

Clear Confidence
2 Drops Geranium
3 Drops Lavender
4 Drops Lime

Concentration Persuasion
2 Drops Brain Power
2 Drops Lemon
2 Drops Clarity

Idea Makers
2 Drops Peppermint
2 Drops Orange
2 Drops Frankincense

Bright Minds
2 Drops Rosemary
2 Drops Orange
2 Drops Peppermint

Achiever Blends
3 Drops Lemon
3 Drops Peppermint

Power Alert
2 Drops Wild Orange
2 Drops Peppermint

Free Flowing
3 Drops Rosemary
2 Drops Lemon

Happy

Lift Me Up
2 Drops Sweet Orange
2 Drops Lemon
2 Drops Bergamot

Celebrate Life!
1 Drop Bergamot
1 Drop Lime
1 Drop Lemon
1 Drop Wild Orange
1 Drop Peppermint

I like to move it
2 Drops Frankincense
2 Drops Peppermint
2 Drops Wild Orange
2 Drops Lime

Crazy Happy
3 Drops Wild Orange
3 Drops Grapefruit
2 Drops Lemon
2 Drops Bergamot

Vivacious
3 Drops Thieves
3 Drops Lemon
3 Drops Frankincense
1 Drops Oregano

Fabulous in a Bottle
3 Drops Bergamot
2 Drops Geranium
1 Drop Sweet Orange
1 Drop Rose

Up Up & Away
3 Drops Bergamot
2 Drops Lavender
2 Drops Clary Sage
1 Drop Ylang Ylang

Happy Indulgence
1 Drop Spruce
1 Drop Cedarwood
1 Drop Juniper Berry
1 Drop White Fir

Your Finest Day
1 Drop Lavender
1 Drop Sweet (Wild) Orange
1 Drop Geranium
1 Drop Clary Sage

Wonderful Joy
3 Drops Bergamot
2 Drops Geranium
3 Drops Lavender

Too Fancy
2 Drops Frankincense
2 Drops Orange
2 Drops Lavender

Wonderfully Made
2 Drops Frankincense
2 Drops Bergamot
2 Drops Orange

Fab Life
4 Drops Orange
2 Drops Lavender
1 Drop Ylang Ylang

Child Wonders
1 Drop Ylang Ylang
2 Drops Sweet (Wild) Orange
1 Drop Lavender

Lift Me Up
2 Drops Sweet Orange
2 Drops Lemon
2 Drops Bergamot

Effervescence
5 Drops Joy
5 Drops Peppermint

Be Gregarious!
4 Drops Bergamot
4 Drops White Angelica

Blues Away!
4 Drops Joy
4 Drops Orange

Festive
2 Drops Joyful Blend
2 Drops Invigorating Blend

Fun-fetti!
3 Drops Grapefruit
2 Drops Fennel

Headache

Think Positive
9 Drops Rosemary
5 Drops Melaleuca
4 Drops Geranium
3 Drops Peppermint
2 Drops Eucalyptus
2 Drops Lavender

Enlighten Your Mind
2 Drops Marjoram
2 Drops Thyme
2 Drops Rosemary
2 Drops Peppermint
2 Drops Lavender

Be Positive
1-2 Drops Marjoram
1-2 Drops Thyme
1-2 Drops Rosemary
1-2 Drops Peppermint
1-2 Drops Lavender

Crave for Peace
2 Drops Sweet Marjoram
2 Drops Thyme
2 Drops Rosemary
2 Drops Peppermint
2 Drops Lavender

Fit Mind

2 Drops Peppermint
2 Drops Lavender
1 Drop Eucalyptus
1 Drop Rosemary

The Comfort Bubble

4 Drops Lavender
4 Drops Peppermint
2 Drops Frankincense
2 Drops Basil

No Jitters

2 Drops Lavender
2 Drops Wild Orange
1 Drop Geranium
1 Drop Clary Sage

No More Headaches!

3 Drops Peppermint
2 Drops Eucalyptus
1 Drops Myrrh

Manifest Healthy Mind

3 Drops Frankincense
3 Drops Lavender
3 Drops Bergamot

The Good Energy
2 Drops Rosemary
2 Drops Peppermint
2 Drops Lavender

Calm the Mind
5 Drops Clove Bud
2 Drops Frankincense
2 Drops Lemon

Change of Pace
5 Drops Lavender
3 Drops Lemongrass
2 Drops Peppermint

Pleasure Seeker
3 Drops Coriander
3 Drops Peppermint
3 Drops Rosemary

Peace Indulgence
3 Drops Lavender
2 Drops Cedarwood
2 Drops Vetiver

Immune System

Immune Power
2 Drops Peppermint
2 Drops Lemon
2 Drops Eucalyptus
1 Drop Rosemary
1 Drop Lime
1 Drop Clove

Instant Booster
2 Drops Lemon
1 Drop Lime
2 Drops Peppermint
1 Drop Rosemary
2 Drops Eucalyptus
1 Drop Clove

Immune Power
2 Drops Peppermint
2 Drops Lemon
2 Drops Eucalyptus
1 Drop Rosemary
1 Drop Lime
1 Drop Clove

Fountain of Health
2 Drops Rosemary
2 Drops Clove
2 Drops Eucalyptus
2 Drops Cinnamon
2 Drops Wild Orange

Cure for Ailments
2 Drops Rosemary
2 Drops Clove
2 Drops Eucalyptus
2 Drops Cinnamon
2 Drops Wild Orange

Shots of Health
1 Drop Rosemary
1 Drop Clove
1 Drop Eucalyptus
1 Drop Cinnamon Bark
1 Drop Wild Orange

Immune Shot
1 Drop German Chamomile
4 Drops Fresh Ginger
1 Drop Cinnamon Bark
4-5 Drops Frankincense

Sick Fighter
1 Drops Fir Needle
1 Drops Juniper
1 Drops Cypress
5 Drops Cedarwood

The Good Remedy
4 Drops On Guard
3 Drops Lemon
2 Drops Oregano

The Immunity Line
5 Drops On Guard
2 Drops Lemon
1 Drop Melaleuca

Immunity Support
2 Drops Lavender
2 Drops Lemon
2 Drops Peppermint

The Health Dispenser
7 Drops On Guard
4 Drops Lemon
2 Drops Melaleuca

Health Pursuit
5 Drops Lavender
2 Drops Geranium
3-4 Drops Rosemary

Health Mobilizer
4 Drops Lemon
4 Drops Grapefruit
2 Drops Oregano

The Cure Station
4 Drops Thieves
4 Drops Purification

Ailment Solution
3 Drops Thieves
3 Drops Purification

Insect Repellent

Bugs Away
4 Drops Spearmint
4 Drops Peppermint
4 Drops Citronella
1 Drop Lemongrass

Shoo Fly
2 Drops Lemongrass
2 Drops Thyme
2 Drops Eucalyptus
2 Drops Basil

Mosquito Go
1 Drop Lemongrass
1 Drop Melaleuca
1 Drop Thyme
1 Drop Eucalyptus
1 Drop Rosemary

Itch Gone
2 Drops Lemon
3 Drops Thieves

Bug Off
3 Drops Lemongrass
3 Drops Citronella

No More Bites
1 Drop Lemongrass
1 Drop Thyme
1 Drop Eucalyptus
1 Drop Basil

Natural Off
3 Drops Lemon Eucalyptus
3 Drops Lavender

Get Away Bug
2 Drops Lavender
2 Drops Geranium
1 Drop Cedarwood

Peace

Harmony in a Bottle
4 Drops Lavender
2 Drops Vetiver

Ohhhhhmmmmmm
2 Drops Lavender
2 Drops Stress Away

Made Like New
4 Drops Purification
1 Drop Lemon
1 Drop Tea Tree

Peaceful Slumber
3 Drops Peace and Calming
2 Drops Valor
1 Drop Lavender

Chakra Peace
2 Drops Lavender
2 Drops Lemon
2 Drops Peppermint

Tranquile Oxidizer
3 Drops Valor
2 Drops Frankincense
1 Drop Lavender

Peaceful Arise
2 Drops Peppermint
2 Drops Orange
2 Drops Lemon

Serenity & Joy
3 Drops Joy
2 Drops Copaiba

Harmony Surround
2 Drops Lavender
2 Drops Lemon
1 Drop Rosemary
1 Drop Peppermint

Peaceful Warrior
3 Drops Frankincense
2 Drops Cedarwood
1 Drop Lemon {or 1 Drop Peppermint}

Let Go and Let Life
3 Drops Bergamot
2 Drops Lemongrass
1 Drops Lemon

Groovy and Wonderful!
2 Drops Tangerine
1 Drop Lemon
1 Drop Lime
1 Drop Grapefruit
1 Drop Orange

World Peace
3 Drops Thieves
3 Drops Citrus Fresh

Refresh

Tropical Wind
3 Drops Grapefruit
3 Drops Lavender
2 Drops Lemon
2 Drops Spearmint

Cool Breeze
4 Drops Spearmint
4 Drops Peppermint
4 Drops Citronella
1 Drop Lemongrass

Freshen Up Your Day
3 Drops Thieves
3 Drops Peppermint

Morning Comfort
3 Drops Bergamot
3 Drops Ylang Ylang

Trail Along the Woods
3 Drops Idaho Balsam Fir
3 Drops Ylang Ylang

Who Runs the World
3 Drops Grapefruit
3 Drops Joy

Back to Young
3 Drops Pan Away
3 Drops Stress Away

Chill in 3 2 1
3 Drops Patchouli
3 Drops Ylang Ylang

Relaxation

Contentment
2 Drops Lavender
3 Drops Purification

Get into the Zone
4 Drops Stress Away
4 Drops Peppermint

Ultimate R & R
2 Drops Copaiba
4 Drops Lavender

Cares Away
5 Drops Lavender
3 Drops Lemongrass

Soothe Balm
4 Drops M-grain
2 Drops Peppermint
2 Drops Lavender

Mind Meditation
3 Drops Patchouli
3 Drops Ylang Ylang

Taming the Storm
2 Drops Lavender
2 Drops Cedarwood
2 Drops Vetiver

After Hours Special
3 Drops Peppermint
3 Drops Lime

It's Easy Time
3 Drops Lavender
3 Drops Bergamot

Back to Sanity
3 Drops Lavender
3 Drops Lime
1 Drop Spearmint

The Comfort Outlet
1 Drop Frankincense
1 Drop Ylang Ylang
1 Drop Sandalwood
1 Drop Patchouli

Redefining Calm
1 Drop Geranium
2 Drops Rose
1 Drop Ylang Ylang

Romance

Romantic Vibe
5 Drops Sandalwood
3 Drops Bergamot
1 Drop Ginger
1 Drop Lime
1 Drop Ylang Ylang

Sexy Smooth
2 Drops Cinnamon
2 Drops Patchouli
1 Drop Rosemary
1 Drop Sandalwood
1 Drop Ylang Ylang

Breathtakingly Sexy
1 Drop Frankincense
1 Drop Geranium
1 Drop Orange
2 Drops Ylang Ylang

Desire & Passion
1 Drop Cedarwood
1 Drop Orange
2 Drops Sandalwood
2 Drops Ylang Ylang

Love Unleashed
3 Drops Ylang Ylang
2 Drops Orange
3 Drops Idaho Blue Spruce

Romantic Way
2 Drops Clary Sage
3 Drops Sensation
2 Drops Idaho Blue Spruce

Sexy Silhouette
1 Drop Jasmine
3 Drops Neroli
2 Drops Rose

Sheer Love
3 Drops Clary Sage
1 Drop Lavender
2 Drops Ylang Ylang

Love Lace
2 Drops Patchouli
1 Drop Orange
4 Drops Ylang Ylang

Captivating Passion
2 Drops Black Pepper
2 Drops Grapefruit
1 Drop Jasmine

Wake Me Up Honey
5 Drops Ylang Ylang
5 Drops Grapefruit

Amorous
3 Drops Goldenrod
3 Drops Sensation

Spark of Desire
4 Drops Idaho Balsam Fir
2 Drops Ylang Ylang

Sound Asleep

Replete & Relaxed
3 Drops Balance
2 Drops Lavender
2 Drops Roman Chamomile
2 Drops Vetiver

Put the Alarm Off
3 Drops Lavender
2 Drops Marjoram
1 Drop Orange
1 Drop Roman Chamomile

The Long Haul
3 Drops Lavender
3 Drops Roman Chamomile
2 Drops Cedarwood
2 Drops Vetiver

Heavenly Peace
4 Drops Lavender
2 Drops Roman Chamomile
2 Drops Sweet Orange
2 Drops Vetiver

Restful Sleep
2 Drops Lavender
2 Drops Sandalwood
2 Drops Chamomile
2 Drops Vetiver

The Slow Lane
3 Drops Juniper Berry
3 Drops Roman Chamomile
3 Drops Lavender

Mellow Blend
3 Drops Vetiver
3 Drops Lavender
2 Drops Frankincense

Hit the Snooze
3 Drops Lemon
3 Drops Lavender
3 Drops Peppermint

Hit the Sack
3 Drops Lavender
3 Drops Wild Orange
3 Drops Roman Chamomile

Break the Busy
2 Drops Copaiba
2 Drops Lavender
2 Drops Stress Away

Sleep like A Child
4 Drops Lavender
2 Drops Cedarwood
2 Drops Gentle Baby

The Sleepy Slope
4 Drops Lavender
2 Drops Cedarwood
4 Drops Valor (optional)

Dear Sleep
2 Drops Valerian
3 Drops Lavender
2 Drops Roman Chamomile

Dreamland
3 Drops Valor
2 Drops RC
2 Drops Lavender

Silent Night
3 Drops Lavender
2 Drops RutaVaLa
2 Drops Roman Chamomile

Sleep Well
2 Drops Lavender
2 Drops Chamomile
2 Drops Vetiver

Yes to Repose
2 Drops Lavender
2 Drops Vetiver
2 Drops Marjoram

Quiet Jungle
3 Drops Roman Chamomile
2 Drops Bergamot
2 Drops Frankincense

State of Calm
3 Drops Grounding Blend
2 Drops Lavender
2 Drops Roman Chamomile

State of Gentleness
2 Drops Lavender
2 Drops Roman Chamomile
2 Drops Marjoram

Night Cap in a Bottle
3 Drops Patchouli
2 Drops Wild Orange
2 Drops Frankincense

Seriously Asleep
3 Drops Vetiver
3 Drops Lavender
2 Drops Frankincense

Hush Baby Sleep
2 Drops Frankincense
2 Drops Cedarwood
2 Drops Chamomile

Cradle Rest
3 Drops Petitgrain
2 Drops Orange
1 Drop Fennel

Nocturnal Buddy
3 Drops Lavender
2 Drops Sandalwood
1 Drop Vetiver

Goodnight Kiss
3 Drops Bergamot
2 Drops Cedarwood
1 Drop Marjoram

Rock to Sleep
2 Drops Cedarwood
2 Drops Orange
2 Drops Lavender

Mother's Cradle
3 Drops Cedarwood
3 Drops Lavender
2 Drops Vetiver

Happy Sleep
3 Drops Lavender
2 Drops Ylang Ylang
1 Drop Chamomile

Deep Sleep
3 Drops Juniper Berry
2 Drops Bergamot
1 Drop Chamomile

Imagine Tranquil
4 Drops Cedarwood
3 Drops Cavender

Nappy Time
4 Drops Cedarwood
3 Drops Lavender

Kids on Hibernation
3 Drops Orange
3 Drops Cedarwood

Both Eyes Shut
3 Drops Vetiver
3 Drops Lavender

Closing Time
3 Drops Lavender
3 Drops Cedarwood

In a State of Trance
3 Drops Bergamot
3 Drops Lavender

8 hours Sleep
3 Drops Lavender
3 Drops Sweet (Wild) Orange

Slumber into Sweet Dreams
3 Drops Lavender
3 Drops Vetiver

Sound Asleep
3 Drops Vetiver
3 Drops Calming Blend

Sleep like a Baby
3 Drops Patchouli
3 Drops Sandalwood

Night Wonders
4 Drops Lavender
3 Drops Bergamot

Lotsa Zzzs
4 Drops Lavender
2 Drops Orange

Stress Relief

Create Normal
4 Drops Lavender
3 Drops Clary Sage
2 Drops Ylang Ylang
1 Drop Marjoram

Zen Relief
4 Drops Lavender
2 Drops Cedarwood
2 Drops Wild Orange
1 Drop Ylang Ylang

Alarm on Snooze
4 Drops Lavender
2 Drops Vetiver
1 Drop Clary Sage
1 Drop Lemon

Chill Pill Blend
4 Drops Cedarwood
3 Drops Bergamot
2 Drops Jasmine
1 Drop Neroli

Positive Experience
4 Drops Lavender
3 Drops Clary Sage
2 Drops Ylang Ylang
1 Drop Marjoram

Shrew off!
2 Drops Vetiver
2 Drops Lavender
2 Drops Sandalwood
2 Drops Cedarwood

Comfort Allure
3 Drops Lavender
2 Drops Roman Chamomile
2 Drops Ylang Ylang

Bounty in Peace
3 Drops Bergamot
3 Drops Frankincense
3 Drops Elevation

Find Solace
3 Drops Bergamot
3 Drops Patchouli
3 Drops Ylang Ylang

Chillaxin
3 Drops Bergamot
3 Drops Frankincense
2 Drops Lemon

Laid Back
2 Drops Patchouli
2 Drops Lavender
3 Drops Sandalwood

Captivating Tranquil
3 Drops Peppermint
2 Drops Grapefruit
2 Drops Rosemary

Unfazed
4 Drops Frankincense
4 Drops Balance

State of Equilibrium
3 Drops Stress Away
3 Drops Lavender

Tame the Storm
2 Drops Frankincense
2 Drops Bergamot

Anxiety Buster

4 Drops Peppermint
2 Drops Grapefruit

Morning Frisk

3 Drops Frankincense
3 Drops Lavender

Workout

Motivate Me Everyday
2 Drops Lemon
2 Drops Peppermint
2 Drops Grapefruit

Electrifying
2 Drops Lavender
2 Drops Jasmine
15 Drops Vanilla

Grit & Nailing It
2 Drops Lavender
2 Drops Sandalwood
1 Drop Chamomile

High Calibre Spirit
4 Drops Grapefruit
4 Drops Lemon
4 Drops Peppermint

Invigorate Me
1 Drop Grapefruit
1 Drop Lemon
1 Drop Orange

Steady and Ready
2 Drops Peppermint
2 Drops Lemon
2 Drops Grapefruit

Power Steady
4 Drops Lemon
3 Drops Lemongrass
3 Drops Eucalyptus
3 Drops Peppermint
2 Drops Marjoram

Ruler of the Pack
2 Drops Peppermint
2 Drops Rosemary
2 Drops Lemon

Posed to Bullseye
3 Drops Peppermint
3 Drops Rosemary
3 Drops Orange

Book Ordering

To order your copy / copies of

Diffusers for
Essential Oils

please visit:
OilNaturalEmpress.com

You can also check out other titles available.

Bulk Pricing and
Affiliate Programs Available

Printed in Great Britain
by Amazon

43774673R00059